Weight Loss Guide & Workbook

DISASTROUS DIETS

Stop Dieting & Start Losing Weight!

LAURA ALVARADO

INMOTION Fitness
1758 Industrial Way Suite 112
Napa, CA 94558

www.inmotionfitstudio com

This book is dedicated
to all my wonderful clients over
the past decade.

Thank you. Without your
continued support, I would have
never achieved my dreams.

Contents

Introduction

I'm Coach Laura. I am a lifestyle coach who helps my clients make positive life changes. I'm here to teach you how to finally lose weight and get your life back!

I wrote this book because I was tired of seeing my friends and family waste their time and money on diets that don't work. I've watched countless clients fall for infomercials and other advertising that promise unrealistic results and cause them to get discouraged when they were not able to lose weight on diets making outlandish claims. Sound familiar?

You're here because something in your life needs to change. The information I'm about to share with you is going to help you become stronger and more resilient, have more confidence, and more energy, decrease stress and ultimately live a happier and more fulfilled life. Are you ready to start this life changing journey?

PART ONE
Disastrous Diets

We've all tried at least one. In fact, most of us have probably tried and failed at a diet a few times....

But I'm here to tell you it's not your fault! Diets are disastrous. The faster results are promised, the quicker you are set up to fail.

Over the past decade as a fitness professional, I have NEVER seen a client succeed long-term on a diet. Period.

Fear not! I have witnessed success. Lots of it. Hundreds of pounds lost and kept off. The secret? Avoid following a specific diet. Diets are impossible to follow for the long haul. Clients who lose weight and keep it off developed new healthy habits they could stick to. They achieved this by making small, incremental changes over time.

In the following pages, you will discover why you have never before been able to lose weight. And, using my proven *Healthy Habits Steps for Success Program,* I will show you the secret to finally lose weight and keep it off for good.

This book is filled with exercises to help you personalize this program, discover what's not working in your life and how to change it. You are a wonderfully unique individual. A one-sized-fits-all program won't work. If you are serious about losing weight, don't skip these exercises!

Start by writing down your weight loss goal:

_____

_____

What will happen once you achieve your goal? How will you feel? How will your life be different?

_____

_____

_____

_____

_____

_____

_____

_____

_____

_____

_____

What will you get out of changing your life?

_____

_____

_____

_____

_____

_____

_____

_____

_____

_____

_____

Where does our nutritional information come from?

First let's take a look at why you probably don't know where to start when it comes to changing your diet.

Look at the list of sources your information on diet and nutrition comes from:

Family
Cultural
Society
Religion
Media
Government "My Plate"
Physician or Health Professional

Make a few notes next to each source and in the margins. What have you learned about eating a healthy diet from each source?

Now look over your notes.   Is all the information the same? If some of the information is different, how do you know which sources to trust?

With so much conflicting information it can be hard to decipher what information is creditable. You already know it's important to eat a healthy diet, but what exactly does that mean?

Popular Diets

There are tons of diets out there.... Atkins, South Beach, Low-Fat, Gluten Free, Zone, Paleo and Raw Food just to name a few. It's hard to know which diet to follow. And to make matters even more confusing the information in popular diets changes over time.

I remember my mom cooking lots of pasta in the 90's. Low fat diets where all the rage. Everyone was loading up on pasta, breads, grains and fat-free foods.

Fast forward a decade and no one eats those foods. Pasta? NEVER! It's all about low-carb. All of a sudden high fat foods are back in style. Pass the bacon please!

But there is one thing that all of these diets have in common: they are restrictive. They work by cutting out one of the macronutrient groups – protein, carbohydrates or fat.

Diet Disaster #1 Eliminating Food Groups

Will giving up all breads, grains and fruits shed pounds quickly? You bet! Are you prepared to give up those foods for the rest of your life? Probably not. Most diets work by eliminating one or more food groups. This just isn't realistic for long periods of time. Instead of eliminating foods altogether, focus on moderation and balance. All foods can be enjoyed as part of a healthy diet. The next time you have dessert, enjoy it! By ditching the guilt associated with eliminating certain foods, you can savor an appropriate serving without the cravings and binges that result from trying to forgo the treat altogether.

How do you feel when you are dieting?

Spend a few moments writing down your experiences while on a diet. How did you feel? What happened?

_____
_____
_____
_____
_____
_____
_____
_____
_____
_____

The Deadly Diet Trap

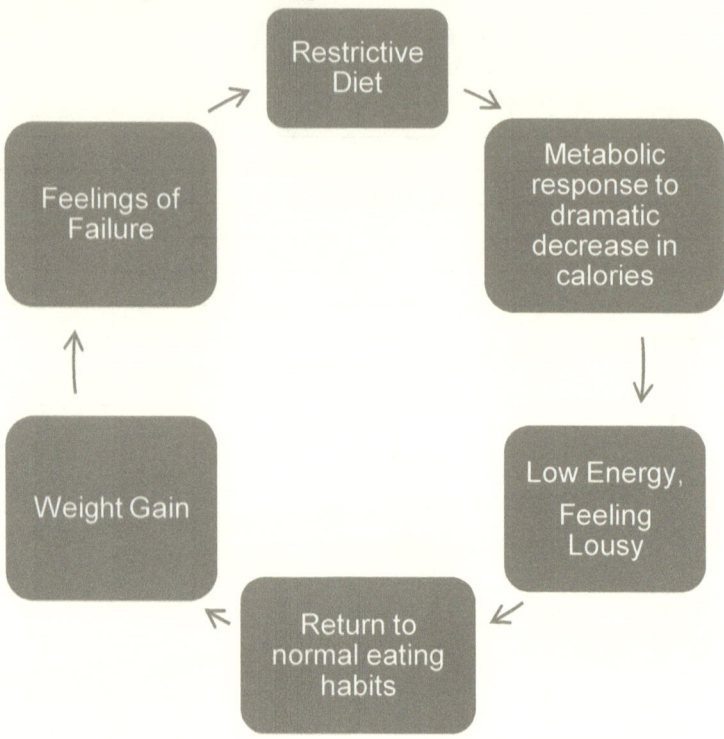

Diets work by removing one of the macronutrients (protein, carbs or fat) and drastically cutting the number of calories you are consuming. Your body responds by going into starvation mode, significantly lowering your metabolism and quickly storing food as fat.

When this happens, you start to experience some of the negative side effects of a restrictive diet. You have intense food cravings, feel lousy and have no energy.

So you return to your old way of eating. Now here is where the problem begins. Even though you return to your 'normal eating habits,' your body is still in starvation mode in response to the restrictive diet. That is why people often gain more weight after a restrictive diet than their pre diet weight.

Diet Disaster #2 Eating Too Few Calories

Have you ever snapped at someone when you are super hungry? Felt drained of energy or moody from low blood sugar? A healthy diet should nourish your body and leave you feeling energized. Over-restricting calories can affect every aspect of your life; not just your waistline. Decreased activity, loss of motivation, difficulty focusing, and inability to regulate stress hormones are all side effects of calorie deprivation. Plus, these diets wreak havoc on your metabolism (this explains why yo-yo dieters gain back more weight after a failed diet attempt). Fuel your body with enough macronutrients to conquer your workday and your next sweat session!

In the deadly diet trap, you set yourself up for failure from the start. Diets don't work because they are too restrictive. Life outside the diet happens (vacation, social commitments, work events or travel) and you can't diet forever – seriously, who wants to cut out carbs for the rest of their life?

How did you feel when you previously abandoned a diet?

_____
_____
_____
_____
_____
_____
_____
_____
_____

You started out hopeful. *This is it. This time I will finally lose weight! This time will be different. I will be stronger and won't give in to temptation.* But then the negative thinking starts...*I am so weak, I can't believe I gave into temptation. I am worthless. No one will love or care about me if I don't lose weight.*

You set yourself up for failure when you choose a diet that is too restrictive and impossible maintain. You inevitably "fail" and eat something that is not allowed on the diet. You beat yourself up. You might as well give up.

This is called *All or Nothing* thinking. It keeps you locked in the deadly diet trap. You are constantly setting yourself up for failure then beating yourself up when it happens. Out of desperation from feeling negatively about yourself, you try yet another restrictive diet. The cycle continues.

Diet Disaster #3 Negative Self Talk

How do you feel when someone constantly puts you down? Does their negativity motivate you? Then why would you constantly put yourself down and expect to be successful? Most of us would never treat someone else the way we treat ourselves. Making change is already challenging enough. Choosing not to criticizing your body and your weight loss efforts is probably the hardest part of losing weight.

So how do I get out of the deadly diet trap?

Letting Go of Guilt!

In order to create new healthy habits, you have to change your thinking. What if I told you from this moment forward you can't eat pizza again, EVER? You might start to think to yourself *"hmm I really want a pizza right now."* You might start to remember how good pizza tastes. Can you picture it in your head right now?

Plain and simple, when you restrict foods, you end up craving them. When you inevitably indulge in those cravings, you feel guilty. *I have already screwed up my diet so I might as well make it worth it!* Now you eat the entire pizza. And maybe some ice cream. You feel even worse, plagued with guilt. You promise yourself you will do better next time.

We already know that diets are disastrous. Instead of focusing on taking away foods, you need to change your thinking

✓ Stop labeling foods as "good" or "bad"

  o Eliminating foods makes them the focus

✓ Stop *stressing* about making poor nutritional choices

  o "All or Nothing" Thinking

✓ Give yourself permission to enjoy food

  o Enjoy all food in moderation

  o Learn what a serving size looks like

Instead of dieting, try focusing on foods that nourish your body, give you energy and make you feel good.

When I take time to eat a hearty breakfast, I am more productive until lunch.

When I eat protein in the afternoon, I have more energy when I get home to spend time with my kids.

What foods can you add to your diet to get to more energy, feel better and have more time for what you love? *Think back to your reasons for wanting to lose weight in the first exercise. Is your current way of eating preventing you from getting what you really want?*

_____

_____

_____

_____

_____

_____

_____

_____

_____

The Power of Quitting
Sometimes it's okay to quit! Yes, you heard me right.

We are taught to never give up; to struggle, push through and to continue on. But refusing to quit an unattainable goal can have detrimental consequences. Here is the typical scenario...

Jane comes in with an unattainable goal. She wants to lose too much weight too quickly for a high school reunion. Jane is determined to stick to a diet that is too strict. The diet eliminates too many food groups and doesn't fit in with her lifestyle.

Jane is able to stick to the diet for a few weeks. She pushes through four challenging spin classes a week. She is having trouble recovering and feels depleted after exercising. Jane is moody and has no energy. She misses going out to dinner with friends because the restaurant doesn't have any options on the menu that fit within the strict guidelines of her diet.

Jane eventually gives up the diet and starts missing spin class. She feels like a failure. Jane is ashamed that she can't lose weight or stick to a diet.

 But Jane was right to quit her extreme weight loss plan. Her goals were unattainable, so she had no chance at being successful. Instead of feeling energized from her workouts, she felt drained. Instead of creating new healthy habits, Jane's diet depleted her body of nutrients.

Setting realistic, attainable goals will make you feel empowered to create positive change in your life. Take a look at the parts of your life that are making you unhappy. Are you sticking around at a job that makes you unhappy because you have invested too much time to quit? Are you unhappy with your health but feel hopeless about making changes because you have previously failed all your attempts to lose weight? *You can choose to be healthy, happy and successful.*

Sometimes that choice includes quitting something in your life that isn't working. Your goals and ambitions may change. *Give yourself permission to quit.* The key is to let go of the fact that you quit, and focus on learning from what went wrong.

S.M.A.R.T .GOALS

Think about what you REALLY want. The best way to get there is to set **S.M.A.R.T. Goals** (Specific, Measurable, Attainable, Realistic, and Time-bound).

Re-examine your previous goal from the first exercise. Is it realistic with everything else you have going on in your life? Measurable (lose some weight vs. lose 5 lbs.)? Is your goal 'someday' or does it have a deadline?

Long Term SMART GOAL

I want to lose 10 lbs by April 15th.

_____
_____
_____
_____

Why do you want to achieve your goal?

I want to have more energy so I can play with my kids.

I want to have more self-confidence so I can feel at ease in social situations and meet new people.

_____
_____
_____
_____
_____
_____
_____
_____

What will happen if you achieve your goal?

My life will be richer if I have more time and energy for family.

I will be happier if I am able to socialize without fear and meet a partner.

_____
_____
_____
_____
_____
_____
_____
_____

How are you going to achieve your goal?

Start by setting smaller goals that are easily attainable in a short period of time. The goals should be realistic for your lifestyle. If you only have 20 minutes in the morning to get ready, no matter how beneficial, cooking eggs for breakfast just isn't a realistic option.

Sub-Goal 1

Jane chooses to drink a glass of water every morning as a way to begin making changes to her diet.

_____
_____
_____
_____

Sub-Goal 2

Jane signs up for 10 sessions with a personal trainer. She knows the accountability of a trainer will help her make going to the gym part of her after work routine.

_____
_____
_____
_____

Sub-Goal 3

Jane always beats herself up about her thighs and compares herself to others in skinny jeans. Jane speaks the same positive affirmation in the mirror every morning, even if she isn't ready to believe it yet. "I love my curvy figure!"

_____
_____
_____
_____

When Jane completes her SMART Goals she feels empowered to make other positive changes to her diet. Soon Jane has achieved lots of sub- goals, has lost a few pounds, and feels great!

In the next chapter you will learn the first step to letting go of guilt, breaking down all of the misleading information on food you have absorbed over the years.

Macronutrients

What are these macronutrients you keep talking about?
Energy Producing Substances

Protein – Carbohydrates - Fat

All foods are made up of macronutrients; protein, carbohydrates and fats. In order to meet your body's nutrient requirements, you will need to eat a large quantity of each macronutrient. Micronutrients are nutrients you need in smaller quantities.

Earlier we learned that most popular diets work by eliminating one of the macronutrients. This can be detrimental to your health because each macronutrient plays an import role in your body.

PROTEINS
Amino Acids "the building blocks"

Proteins are comprised of 20 amino acids. There are 8 essential amino acids that cannot be manufactured in the body. You will need to get these from the foods you eat.

Each amino acid is needed for optimum health. If you eat a diet that is deficient in one or more amino acids, certain proteins will not be made and the function that protein carries out in your body will be lost.

Essential amino acids can be found in both animal and plant food sources. Complete proteins contain all essential amino acids. Generally, animal products are complete protein sources such as eggs, meat or fish. Plants typically contain some but not all of the essential amino acids. Vegetarians and vegans need to eat a variety of plant proteins to ensure essential amino acid needs are met.

FAT
"Eating fat will make you FAT"

Just like there are essential amino acids, there are essential fatty acids that your body cannot produce. These fatty acids are necessary for many functions throughout the body such as brain and heart health. Fats are also important for the absorption of fat-soluble vitamins.

It's a common misconception that eating fat will make you fat. Don't confuse the fat in your food with the fat in your body.

There are three main types of fats; unsaturated (monounsaturated and polyunsaturated), saturated and trans fats. Generally unsaturated fats come from plants and saturated fats are found in animal products. Trans fats are artificial and should be avoided.

Make a list of foods you tend to reach for when you are famished:

_____
_____
_____
_____
_____
_____
_____
_____
_____

Look at your list. Most of us go for convenience foods, typically foods higher in sugar. **Circle these foods.**

Sugar is quickly turned into glucose. This causes a quick rise in blood sugar levels and makes you hungry again sooner. Spikes and crashes in your blood sugar levels lead to spikes and crashes in your energy.

Conversely fat slows down the breakdown absorption process of food keeping you feeling fuller longer. Remember feeling hungry all the time on your last diet? Hunger is a huge reason why most diets don't work. The most important thing to remember about fat is that it aids in satiety or "feeling full."

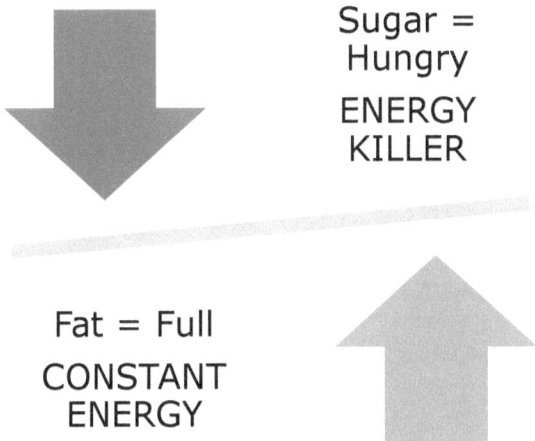

Sugar =
Hungry
ENERGY
KILLER

Fat = Full
CONSTANT
ENERGY

So the next time you're feeling ravenous choose a nutrient dense, fatty food. Some options include nuts and seeds, avocado, full fat dairy products, fish and egg yolks.

Make a list of some of the high nutrient fatty foods you enjoy:

_____
_____
_____
_____
_____
_____

CARBOHYDRATES
"Everything Else"

Carbohydrates are in everything from fruit, vegetables, grains, beans, dairy nuts and seeds to the more commonly thought of bread and pasta. You might think of carbs as that evil bread group in the food pyramid but the truth is most of the foods we eat have some amount of carbohydrates in them.

Carbohydrates can be broken down into three categories; starch, sugar and fiber. Complex carbohydrates have more fiber. Simple carbohydrates don't. Just like fat, fiber slows down your digestive process. Therefore, simple carbohydrates should be enjoyed in moderation.

Simply put carbohydrates are energy. In fact, they are your body's main source of energy (glucose). You are not going to stick to a diet if you feel sluggish all the time. And if you forgo carbs altogether you are likely to crave the fastest and easiest source, sugar. Adding high fiber foods to your diet will help ward off unwanted sugar cravings and fuel your body with enough energy to knock out your to-do list.

Creating Healthy Habits

We are creatures of habit. Much like the rest of your life, the way we eat is based on a series of habits. These habits can come from necessity, convenience, tradition, or are culturally or religious based. Habits are created over time. You have to repeat the same action over and over again for it to become a habit.

People who want quick, immediate change often end up trying to change too many things at once. When this doesn't work, they revert back to their old habits.

Diet Disaster #4 Unrealistic Change

The key to losing weight and keeping it off is to establish new healthy habits. In order to become a habit, an action has to be repeated over and over again. This takes time. And so will losing weight. Focusing on changes that are too drastic, don't fit your lifestyle, or trying to change too many habits at once is a recipe for failure.

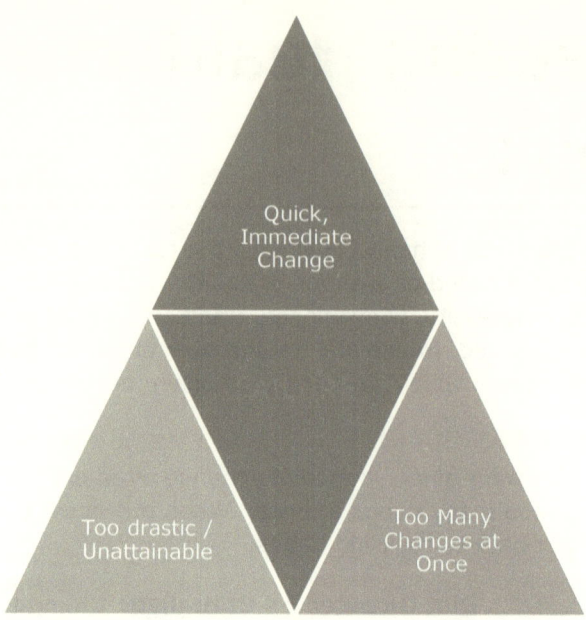

Start by focusing on a single action; something easy to incorporate into your current lifestyle such as drinking 8 glasses of water daily. Focus all your attention on that single action until it becomes a healthy habit. Then move onto another habit. When you are successful, congratulate yourself. Making change is hard!

Start with change that is easily made. When you are able to be successful from the beginning changing further actions will be easy. When you try to make unrealistic change and fail, feelings of hopelessness will make your future weight loss attempts more challenging.

PART TWO
STEPS TO SUCCESS

Finally, the part you have been waiting for. A decade of helping people just like you make lasting and meaningful life changes has produced these sure fire steps to success.

Before you get started on your life transformation, remember:

- ✓ Achieve success by focusing all your attention on a single step

- ✓ Choose small, manageable steps that you can start taking TODAY!

- ✓ **Don't Rush It!** Don't move on to the next step until your current focus becomes habit

STEP 1 DRINK MORE WATER

Drinking up will boost your metabolism and help prevent you from overeating. It seems easy but you probably aren't drinking enough water. *Exactly how much water should I be drinking?*

STEP GOAL:

WOMEN 3 liters	MEN 4 liters

It's crucial that you are able to be successful with this first step. Success builds upon itself. It's like a snowball, gaining momentum the more you are able to conquer. Choose a goal that fits with your lifestyle. You might want to break this step down into multiple sub-goals. You have a hectic work and social schedule. If drinking 3-4 liters of water daily seems overwhelming, start with something manageable like drinking a glass of water in the morning after you brush your teeth (piggy backing a new habit on an existing one will make it easier).

Sub-goals in this step can include:

- Purchasing a 3-liter bottle and keeping it at your desk to sip on throughout the day
- Reducing consumption of juice, soda and sports drinks
- Drinking water with meals

- Reducing consumption of alcohol
- Giving up diet sodas
- "Hydrate before you caffeinate" - kick starting metabolism by drinking 16oz of water with lemon upon waking
- Keeping pitchers of flavored water on hand in the fridge by adding fresh fruit, lemon or cucumber
- Limiting coffee intake to 1 cup daily or switch to tea

Coffee

Drinking coffee may temporarily give you more energy. Most people don't realize that over-use of coffee can strain on your body's ability to regulate hormones and depletes your body of vitamins and minerals. All of those nasty caffeine side effects are actually going to lower your energy and mess with your body's fat burning abilities.

As you move through your sub-goals, you may find that other parts of your routine need to change in order to make changes to your diet. Do you relax at the end of the day by drinking a beer or a glass of wine? That glass of wine (or two) may be what's stopping you from losing weight. Alcohol may cause you to overeat at dinner and/or make poor food choices. Or simply add too many empty calories. If you are serious about losing weight and keeping it off for good, you will have to find another way to unwind. Sometimes creating a new healthy habit that doesn't involve food can have huge impact on your diet.

What's preventing you from achieving your sub-goals?

I need to find a healthy way to unwind after work, but I don't have enough energy do to anything besides sit on the couch with a beer.

I'm constantly on the go and don't have time to think about drinking water.

Brainstorm new healthy habits to replace barriers

Replace beer with a 10-minute meditation from YouTube on the couch. Relax with a home facial. Sign up for a fitness class after work – get a friend to sign up too so I will actually show up.

Drink more water in the morning before my hectic day starts. Keep a case of water at my desk or a bottle in my car. Set an alarm on my phone or computer to remind me to drink more water. Ask my assistant to bring me water throughout the day instead of coffee.

Circle new habits that are manageable or that seem easy.

Create a list of sub-goals. Start with the easier or less daunting ones at the top and the harder ones towards the bottom.

Don't stress if this list seems long. Remember that once you tackle the smallest goal, the rest will come easier.

_____

_____

_____

_____

_____

_____

_____

_____

_____

STEP 2 NUTRIENT DENSE FOODS

How often do you eat 6-8 servings of fruits and vegetables in a day? Fruits and vegetable supply your body with many important nutrients and are packed full of satiety stimulating fiber.

Your goal in this step is to focus on *adding* instead of *restricting*. The more nutritious foods you eat, the less you will want high-calorie/low nutrition foods (junk food). We want to avoid the diet trap of saying *"I want this but I can't have it."* Instead of classifying foods as "good" or "bad," focus on adding high nutrition foods into your diet.   If your plate is filled with fruits and vegetables, there won't be much room left for foods that should be enjoyed in moderation.

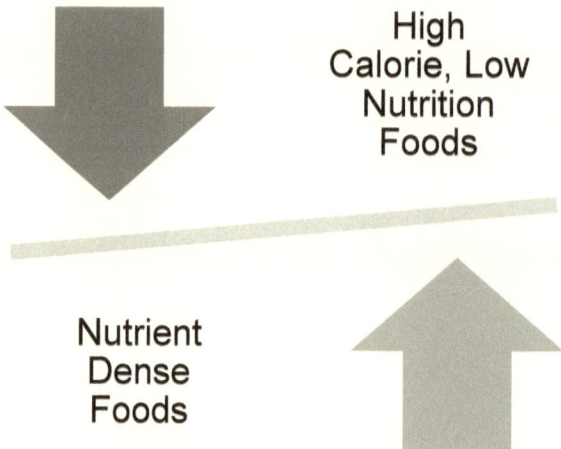

High Calorie, Low Nutrition Foods

Nutrient Dense Foods

STEP GOAL: Add in two servings fruits or vegetables to every meal (breakfast-lunch-dinner). This will give you 6 out of 6-8 recommended daily servings.

Here are a few examples of what your day might look like.

Breakfast

- Adding tomato slices to toast with cheese with a piece of fruit on the side
- Vegetable omelet with 1cup spinach and 1cup mixed veggies such as mushroom and zucchini

Lunch

- Side salad and fruit piece with sandwich or soup
- Large salad (2 cups min) with meat and seeds

Dinner

- Main dish plus two vegetable side dishes (1 cup each) such as roasted winter veggies and kale/dried cherry salad
- Main dish plus dinner side salad and a cup of berries for dessert

Just like in Step One, you may need to break this goal down into sub-goals. Remember we want *realistic* and *manageable* goals.

What's preventing you from achieving this step goal?

I don't have time to prepare all those vegetables.

Brainstorm new healthy habits to replace barriers

Purchase prepared vegetables such as vegetable trays, cut melon, pre-made salads or frozen vegetables. Have fresh fruits delivered to my office.

_____
_____
_____
_____
_____
_____
_____
_____
_____

Possible Step 2 Sub-Goals:

- Make extra food at dinner time and packing leftovers for lunch the next day
- Try a new vegetable each week from the grocery store or famer's market
- Compile a list or restaurants near my office that have lots vegetable items on the menu
- Place a fruit bowl on my desk for healthy snacks at arm's reach
- Prepare five salads in Tupperware on Sunday for the week

-

List Your Step 2 Sub-goals:

Create a list of sub-goals. Start with the easier or less daunting ones at the top and the harder ones towards the bottom.

Don't stress if this list seems long. Remember once you tackle the smallest goal, the rest will come easier.

_____

_____

_____

_____

_____

_____

_____

_____

_____

_____

STEP 3 EAT MORE OFTEN

Most of us don't eat often enough because we are either too busy or believe that if we eat less now, we can eat more later.

How do you feel when you have not eaten all day?

_____
_____
_____
_____
_____
_____
_____
_____

Not eating often enough will not only slow down your metabolism, but will also lower your energy and leave you feeling mentally foggy and irritable. The less energy you have, the less likely you will be able to participate in physical activity or spend time doing the things you love instead of watching TV.

What types of foods do you eat when are really hungry and have low energy?

_____
_____
_____
_____
_____
_____
_____

These are generally high sugar, convenience foods or caffeinated products. When we are starving, we make poor food choices and are more likely to overeat or binge on food.

Your main focus this step is to let go of your fear about eating often. Make intentional, nourishing food choices, keep your metabolism running at its peak, and have tons of energy by eating every 3-4 hours.

STEP GOAL: Enjoy meals or snacks every 3-4 hours

Snack = (Fruit, Vegetable or Starch) + FAT or PROTEIN

- Hard-boiled egg with a piece of fruit
- Baby carrots & hummus
- Celery & peanut butter
- Apple with a slice of cheddar cheese
- Whole grain crackers & string cheese
- 2 TBS almonds and a banana
- Greek yogurt and fruit
- Tuna and whole wheat tortilla
- Figs and brie cheese
- Veggies and guacamole
- Brown rice cakes and PB
- Edamame and baby carrots
- Baked tofu and raw vegetables
- Sliced tomatoes and mozzarella cheese

What is preventing you from achieving this goal?

_____
_____
_____
_____
_____
_____
_____
_____
_____
_____

Brainstorm new healthy habits to replace barriers

_____
_____
_____
_____
_____
_____
_____
_____

Top 5 Healthy Snacks Available Anywhere!

1. **Nuts or Trail Mix** - avoid mixes with added sugar such as candy
2. **Cereal** - look for whole grain, high fiber cereals available at most gas stations. Scan the shelves for whole grain crackers to pair with dairy for a balanced snack
3. **Dairy** - when you stop to fill up your car, check the refrigerated section for string cheese or low-fat yogurt
4. **Fruit** - whole fruit is best, check dried fruit labels for added sweeteners
5. **Bars** - while whole foods are always preferable to processed ones, skip the drive through and grab a high fiber bar to tide you over

Possible Step 3 Sub-Goals:

- Purchase single serving items such as string cheese, individual trail mix packs or yogurts to grab on the go
- Divide boxes of crackers into single servings zip lock bags when I get home from the grocery store
- Make a list of non-perishable snacks I can store at my desk, keep in my purse or car such as bars, protein drinks or trail mix

Create a list of sub-goals. Start with the easier or less daunting ones at the top and the harder ones towards the bottom.

Don't stress if this list seems long. Remember once you tackle the smallest goal, the rest will come easier.

_____
_____
_____
_____
_____
_____
_____

STEP 4 EAT THE RIGHT BREAKFAST

Breakfast. The most important meal of the day. So why do we typically skip breakfast or to grab an unhealthy one like a donut? The answer is probably a lack of time. In fact, most Americans rarely stop their busy lives to eat throughout the day. By the time you get home, you are starving. You consume one large meal then sit in front of the TV drained of energy from your hectic day. Sound familiar?

What does your typical breakfast look like?

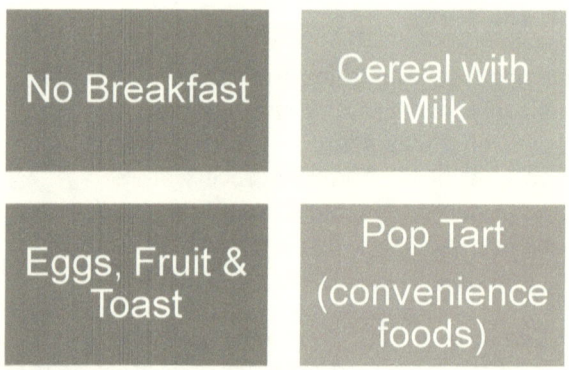

Which of the breakfasts listed above do you think is the best choice?

Eating the right breakfast will help you maintain energy, make better food choices throughout the day, and resist over-eating. This is because breakfast sets insulin sensitivity for the rest of the day. Eating a protein rich breakfast prevents spikes and crashes in blood sugar later in the day, allowing your body to metabolize fat instead of relying so much on sugar.

On the other hand, eating a high sugar / high starch breakfast such as a coffee shop pastry causes an insulin rush. This insulin rush causes your insulin, blood sugar and blood fat levels to remain high for the rest of the day. By pairing starches with fiber, you can slow down their breakdown/absorption process for a more constant supply of energy. (Hyman, M.D., *Ultra-Metabolism*)

Simply put, all this means that eating a breakfast high in protein and fiber is going to give you lasting energy and help you maintain a healthy weight.

STEP 4 GOAL: eat a protein rich breakfast and pair starches with fiber to slow down their breakdown/absorption process.

Breakfast = 2 Fruits or Vegetables + PROTEIN+ FIBER (5g min.)

High Fiber Foods

- Beans
- whole grains
- vegetables
- fruits
- nuts
- seeds

Let's take a look at some examples of high protein, high fiber breakfast combinations.

Optimal Breakfast Combinations

- Oatmeal topped with nuts/seeds and berries
- 2 egg omelet with seasonal veggies and fruit salad
- Whole grain toast with PB and a banana
- Whole grain breakfast sandwich with eggs, tomato and spinach
- Breakfast burrito with 2 eggs, 1/4 c. salsa and 1 c. spinach
- Greek yogurt with 1 c. fresh berries & slivered almonds, cucumber slices
- Whole-grain English muffin with melted cheese & tomato slices, piece of fruit
- Car breakfast: 2 Hard-boiled eggs, banana, baby carrots

What is preventing you from achieving this goal?

_____

_____

_____

_____

_____

_____

_____

_____

_____

_____

Brainstorm new healthy habits to replace barriers

_____

_____

_____

_____

_____

_____

_____

_____

_____

_____

Possible Step 4 Sub-Goals:

- Research a few recipes I can make in advance to save time in the morning like overnight oats or freezing homemade breakfast burritos
- Commit to turning technology off by 9:30PM and going to bed by 10PM so I am able to get up in time for breakfast in the morning.
- Find a coffee shop that has an item on the menu that will fit within my guidelines
- Buy a mini fridge for my office and load it up with hard boiled eggs and Greek yogurt

Create a list of sub-goals. Start with the easier or less daunting ones at the top and the harder ones towards the bottom.

Don't stress if this list seems long. Remember once you tackle the smallest goal, the rest will come easier.

_____
_____
_____
_____
_____
_____
_____
_____
_____
_____

STEP 5 RAID YOUR KITCHEN

Processed Foods - Dump the Junk!

Inherently your body knows how to maintain a healthy weight. Modern day "food" interrupts many of your body's processes and can send mixed signals that cause foods to be stored as fat instead of used for energy.

Take artificial sweeteners as an example. Aspartame may be a popular diet food additive, but it actually cues your body to store fat. Aspartame's sweet taste stimulates appetite and increases sugar cravings. In fact, you are more likely to overeat after consuming artificial sweeteners. You'd be better off chowing down on table sugar than eating artificial sweeteners.

It's pretty scary to think of all the synthetic materials and hormones we dump into our bodies as "food." To think that these additives don't have an effect on your body's ability to produce energy and maintain a healthy weight is foolish. If you want to metabolize more fat and start feeling better, you have to start eating more whole foods.

Go through your pantry and start reading some labels. Use Michael Pollan's guide for determining if you should keep an item or toss it.

Is this packaged Item a WHOLE FOOD item?

    ✓ Are there five ingredients or less?
    ✓ Can I pronounce each of the ingredients?
    ✓ Would my grandmother recognize each
ingredient?
    ✓ Can I find these ingredients in my kitchen?
(Pollan 2008)

*If you answered "no" to any of these questions, you have a processed item. For a better choice, see if you can find a similar item that meets the above criteria.

Eat organic when possible purchasing the highest quality foods that you can afford. Remember, we want to avoid classifying foods as "good" or "bad." Focus on the quality of the ingredients and putting high-nutrition foods into your meals rather than food-like processed products. Go ahead and eat some pizza...can you make the pizza at home using high quality whole foods rather than purchasing a frozen or fast food pizza?

List your favorite processed or diet foods in the right hand column. Make a list of whole food alternatives on the left hand side of the page.

Processed Foods: **Whole Food Alternatives:**

Sugar free candy   *Dark chocolate*

Dorritos   *Kettle chips*

STEP 5 GOAL: Your mission is to raid your kitchen. Eliminate foods containing trans fats, MSG, high fructose corn syrup, and aspartame. Go through your pantry and start reading labels. Use the guidelines above to determine if you should keep an item or throw it away. Start filling up those trash bags! Or donate unopened foods to charity.

STEP 6 MAKE IT EASY – MAKE A PLAN

What is currently preventing you from completing the previous five steps? Look back at the barriers you listed on the previous pages.

The excuse I hear the most often is that people simply don't have time to make better food choices. In most cases some simple planning can solve this problem. Planning meals in advance and shopping from a list will not only help you save time and money at the store, it can also reduce cooking time during the week.   Pick a weekly shopping day and prepare foods when you get home from the store.

How many times have you opened the fridge, stared at a melon or head of broccoli and thought to yourself it's just too much work to wash and cut up?

Wash and cut produce when you get home from the store. Use Tupperware or plastic storage bags to make single serving grab-and-go healthy snacks. You can also save time by purchasing prepared food items like pre-washed and cut vegetables, roasted chicken and frozen produce.

- ✓ Create a weekly meal plan and shopping list
- ✓ Schedule time to prepare items
- ✓ Purchase prepared foods
- ✓ Portion servings in advance

Shopping Guide

Save time in the store by grouping together similar items when you are creating your shopping list.

FRUITS / VEGETABLES

BREAD / GRAINS

DAIRY

MEAT / PROTIEN

BULK / CANNED

Use the menu planning worksheet below to plan meals for the week. Get everything you need for the week in one trip to the store. Save time cooking during the week by planning menus that re-use the same ingredients. For example, cook five chicken breasts at once and use during the week:

1. Chicken dinner with roasted root vegetables
2. Sliced chicken breast on Cobb salad for lunch
3. Diced chicken and black bean tacos for dinner
4. Chicken, egg, spinach and feta omelet breakfast
5. Chicken salad sandwich for lunch

Menu Planning Worksheet

Fill in each meal for the week. Remember your goal is to eat every 3-4 hours. Depending on the time you eat breakfast for example, you may or may not need a morning snack.

Most people eat similar foods each day. You don't need to have five different breakfast options. Even if your breakfast or mid-morning snack is the same each day, write it down and make sure you get enough food at the store for each weekday.

	Monday	Tuesday	Wednesday	Thursday	Friday
Breakfast					
Snack					
Lunch					
Snack					
Dinner					
Dessert					

More Veggies, Less Time!

We all know it's important to eat our vegetables. But let's face it, just the thought of pre-heating an oven and preparing all those yummy vegetables after a long day of work can be tiring.

What's the answer? Drastically cut down cooking time on week nights by pre-roasting all of your vegetables for the week on Sunday.

On the menu this week is curry roasted cauliflower, Italian potatoes, sweet cinnamon carrots and Brussel sprouts.

SUNDAY

Preheat oven to 400 degrees. Wash and trim vegetables. Organize baking sheets and season. Bake vegetable sheets for 20-25 minutes, potatoes sheet for 40 minutes. Mixing trays half way.

Sheet 1: head of cauliflower, 3-4 chopped carrots, half yellow onion, generous covering of each (curry powder, onion powder, garlic powder, chili powder), oil, salt & pepper to taste.

Sheet 2: small potatoes, 3-4 minced cloves garlic, Italian seasoning, oil, salt & pepper to taste.

Sheet 3: Half tray: Brussels sprouts, 1-2 minced cloves garlic, oil, salt & pepper to taste – **Half tray:** whole carrots, generous covering of each (cinnamon & nutmeg), oil, honey, salt & pepper to taste

MONDAY

Mix cauliflower sheet with a can of garbanzo beans and ¼ cup raisins. Serve with rice or quinoa and a simple mixed green salad.

TUESDAY

Heat your favorite sausage and serve with brussel sprouts and potatoes.

WEDNESDAY

Pan sauté chicken breast or tofu in favorite bottled Indian sauce. Mix cinnamon carrots with ¼ cup cashews and chopped parsley. Serve with rice.

*Reserve a few carrots for Thursday

THURSDAY

Nicoise Salad – top a large field of greens with potatoes, hard-boiled egg (boil eggs on Sunday and use all week for healthy snacks), canned tuna, olives, roasted carrots, and fresh vegetables such as tomato, cucumber or avocado. Mix with oil and vinegar dressing.

STEP 7 POSITIVE AFFIRMATIONS

Breaking Down Negative Self talk with Positive Affirmations

How do you feel when someone constantly puts you down? Does their negativity motivate you? Then why would you constantly put yourself down and expect to be successful?

Most of us would never treat someone else the way we treat ourselves. Making change is already challenging enough. Choosing not to criticize your body and your weight loss efforts is probably the hardest part of losing weight.

Changing your inner voice will help you take back the power you have given to food. The biggest obstacle to overcome when creating new healthy habits around food is to separate food from emotion. Are you eating because you are hungry or are you lonely? Bored? Stressed out?

Deciding to change the way you eat will force you to take a look at the role food plays in your life. Food is an integral part of culture. Food should nourish you and provide you with energy, but often it is used for more than that. Healthy traditions around meals are important. Food unites us with friends and family. It can be part of celebrations and traditions. Food can also be used to distract you from unwanted and uncomfortable emotions. If you do not address those emotions, change your thinking and replace food with positive, healthy alternatives, you will never be successful with the six previous steps.

Best practices and questions to ask yourself at mealtime:

- ✓ Focus on enjoying food while you eat. Sit at the table with technology put away. Enjoy mealtime with loved ones whenever possible.
- ✓ Spend at least 30 minutes eating meals. Don't rush.
- ✓ Ask yourself before you eat, 'What am I feeling right now?'
- ✓ Not sure if you are hungry or bored? Drink a glass of water. Wait 10 minutes. 'Am I still hungry?'
- ✓ Incorporate favorite treats (in moderation) into meal plan. If they are in your plan, you are less likely to feel guilty when eating them or to binge on them.

STEP 7 GOAL: Start each day with a positive affirmation. Something you want to change about how you see yourself. At the start of EVERY day look in the mirror and state your positive affirmation out loud. Even if you don't accept or believe it, keep saying it. I guarantee your view will change over time and you will be healthier, happier and more successful!

What areas of your body do you want to change the most? What do you dislike the most about yourself? Use these as a starting off point for positive affirmations.

_____

_____

_____

_____

_____

_____

_____

_____

_____

Turning a negative into a positive

I am constantly using this exercise with my weight loss coaching clients. When my clients are struggling with change and begin to list off everything they are doing wrong, I remind them of what they are doing right. Making change is hard!

- ✓ When you make a mistake, remind yourself of all the positive changes you have already made
- ✓ Don't beat yourself up for something that happened in the past
- ✓ Ask yourself what you are proud of?
- ✓ Use setbacks as a chance to examine what isn't working and to identify barriers for change

Client Jane: "I have been really bad this week. I didn't eat any of my snacks. I was too busy to exercise. I just don't know what's wrong with me. I want to lose weight, but I just can't seem to change anything!"

Me: "How long have you been skipping meals and living a sedentary lifestyle?"

Jane: "A long time. I haven't exercised regularly since college. Ever since I had my kids 10 years ago, I'm just too busy to eat."

Me: "It sounds like you have been engaging in your current habits for over a decade. New habits take time and it's unfair to beat yourself up when things don't change overnight. What did you do differently this week?"

Jane: "I was able to drink my water almost every day."

Me: "And I see from your food journal that you have been eating breakfast consistently for the past three weeks! You have made two new healthy habits. I'm proud of you! It seems like making time for snacks is challenging for you. What can you keep in your purse for a healthy snack on the go?"

Jane: " I like Kind bars. I think they are a whole food."

Me: "Great! Your goal for this week is to order a box from Amazon and keep a few in your purse, office and car."

Turn a Negative into a Positive Exercise

Start with what went right...
Name two things you have accomplished recently you are proud of?

_____
_____
_____
_____
_____
_____
_____
_____
_____

Write down at least one positive change you have made in the past month.

_____
_____
_____
_____
_____
_____
_____
_____
_____

Looking at what went wrong...
You didn't fail because something is wrong with you or because you are weak willed. Understanding why you were not able to change is an important part of letting go of guilt and finding manageable changes.

What change were you trying to make?

_____
_____
_____
_____
_____
_____
_____
_____
_____

Why were you not able to make it?

_____
_____
_____
_____
_____
_____
_____
_____
_____

Identify the barrier

_____
_____
_____
_____
_____
_____
_____
_____
_____

What can you do differently in the future to break down your barriers for change?

_____

_____

_____

_____

_____

_____

_____

_____

_____

Simple Formula for Success

If you take nothing else away from this book remember this simple formula for success:

- ✓ Acknowledge when you do something right
- ✓ Throw out negative self-talk when you make a mistake
- ✓ Instead, figure out what went wrong
- ✓ Come up with a manageable solution

Losing weight is about making life changes, not about dieting. If you truly want to lose weight and keep it off, prepare for the long and rewarding journey ahead.

Be realistic about how long it will actually take you to achieve your weight loss goals. Don't rush the process. Avoid making changes that are too drastic or trying to change too many things at once.

If you are willing to commit to the steps laid out for you in this life changing program, the results will be greater than you ever imagined. Not only will be finally be able to maintain a healthy weight, you will also discover a more balanced, fulfilled and happy lifestyle.

Have questions? Need more assistance in your weight loss efforts? Contact the author at info@inmotionfitstudio.com

www.ingramcontent.com/pod-product-compliance
Lightning Source LLC
Chambersburg PA
CBHW020407290526
45785CB00005B/2465